T0116858

The TRUE Face of Health Care Reform

A Physician and Patient's Perspective

P.Y. Sun, M.Div., M.D.

authorHOUSE®

AuthorHouse™
1663 Liberty Drive
Bloomington, IN 47403
www.authorhouse.com
Phone: 1-800-839-8640

First published by AuthorHouse 10/04/2011

ISBN: 978-1-4567-2135-0 (ebk)
ISBN: 978-1-4567-2134-3 (sc)
ISBN: 978-1-4567-2136-7 (hc)

Library of Congress Control Number: 2011901908

Printed in the United States of America

This book is printed on acid-free paper.

Certain stock imagery © Thinkstock.

Dedication:
To the true teachers who have taught me to care, not in order to receive, but in order to be the Image of our great Physician.

Preface:
(2004)

One month ago, I was going along on my merry way with the rest of the medical residents in pathology, choosing a subspecialty fellowship to train in, when once again the competing interests of patient care and administration interrupted. As a medical fellow, one duty I was responsible for was assessing emergency requests for blood products, determining necessity and best course of action, and possibly authorizing the product release. One call came where the clinical floor and the laboratory were in disagreement as to the best course of action. Following the incident, the medical administrative director stated that the proper response to the call was, "don't ask questions, just give the product." In other words, don't think or diagnose, as our current 9 years: 4 years medical/graduate school and then 5 years of pathology training had taught us, but rather give in to the market and legal forces, and make a blanket sale.

Contents

INTRODUCTION

You hear the horror stories of a surgeon operating on the wrong leg, or side of the body. So far, I've had at least two dentists look at the wrong side of my mouth. The first really seemed to be sleepwalking (are the rumours of self-anesthetizations for dentists true?) Right after examining me, he ordered a dental x-ray– on the wrong side.

The second time a dentist examined the wrong side of my mouth happened recently (2006). On a follow-up visit, after an extensive discussion of my RIGHT upper molar, the dentist re-examined the x-ray taken *in his office*, clearly spelled out "Right" and "Left." He proceeded to talk about how the root canal had not been done well, and then pointed to the LEFT side of my teeth. First, I have had only, thanks be to the Holy Lord God, <u>one</u> root canal. Second, the tooth had been extracted, and had a clear area of greater lucency, as well and area of bone atrophy where the tooth had been. Third, he had just examined that tooth.

Flashback to a renowned Oral Maxillary Facial surgeon, a dentist at a top medical center. (As an indication of the demand for him, the dentist accepts only cash payments.) After multiple visits, it was decided to just extract the tooth. This decision came after the initial root canal, and:

A. the crown broke the next day;

B. the crown was removed two days post placement;

C. three endondontic procedures where a hole was dug in the middle of the tooth again; and

D. two apicoectomies* when a hole the size of a dime was made to my upper jaw, two times because the dental surgeon ignored the root from which the infection was coming.

In short, I had had a raging infection about three inches from my <u>brain</u> for the last 7 years!

Back to the tooth extraction. The dentist jiggled and wiggled the tooth, and I wondered if this was part of the standard process. Finally he said, "I'm just trying to get this crown off." I replied, "There is no crown." The dentist had been pulling at the wrong tooth.

Another caveat came from the same dental surgeon during the initial visit when he prescribed the antibiotic Clindamycin, until Computer Assisted Tomography or CAT scans of my tooth could be taken. I asked him how long I should take the medicine, and he replied, "as long as the tooth hurts," clearly differing from the recommended lengths for efficacy and reduction of resistant bacterial strains. As an explanation, he stated that pretty much the "teeth heal by themselves." I wondered why I was in his office.

*Apicoectomy: A dental procedure in which the roots or apices of the tooth are removed. It was explained to me by a dentist that root canals are not able to be cleaned all the way to the tips of the roots.

THE STATE OF OUR HEALTH CARE

Most people would agree with the statement that our medical care is in need of reform. The high costs, unsatisfactory service, and the loss of human interactions can be seen throughout the industry. As a physician and a patient, I know. I had lived with a raging infection for 7 years in my face–an area that somehow fell between anyone's expertise. The M.D.s said it was the domain of the dentists. A top oral surgeon said, "most things in the teeth heal by themselves." Yet as attested by the lucrative salaries that dental surgeons derive from procedures, the oral surgeon's opinion doesn't seem to be the opinion of most dentists. In my case, a multitude of dental procedures had been performed.

I would like to propose a new way of looking at Health Care. As a physician, I must rally for the practitioners with the central knowledge and practice to be Executives or captains of the medical care ship. Health Care may be viewed through many lenses, but is it logical to have attorneys steering the ship? Would the seamen or medical administrators who make up seaway codes, tucked away in their offices, be the best captains for conditions of storm? How about the medical academicians? Would they be able to judge the best route while at sea or while in the laboratory? Who is the Executive that has the experience of hands-on weathering of storms and complications, with the help of her crewmen (nurses, technicians, therapists)?

Our American history contains the seeds of wisdom that our ancestors established in creating the balance of powers for our governmental system. We have the Executive branch, which is represented by our President. The Legislative branch gives form to the wishes of the people in the structure of laws. The Judicial branch interprets the laws when there are times of disagreement. We can recapture the wisdom of this system by applying the concept of a balanced system of powers to the medical system.

A second misconception of roles is that Health Care has become "consumerized." Health Care has become a commodity, as if Health were the same as a pair of shoes or a new flat-screen TV. While this may work for material objects, the crucial part of the healing process has always been the Patient-Physician Relationship. In fact, many people try to romanticize inanimate objects, referring to cars/boats/planes as "she," in order to fulfill the universal need for relationships.

In any relationship, there are times when two or more people have differing opinions. The differing opinions may be handled differently depending on the roles and the context of the group. Is the primary role the patient-physician relationship? Is it the differing opinions within in a medical team? Is it the differences due to the differing goals of the Executive, Legislative, or Judicial branches of medicine...

Which leads us into the murky waters of conflicts of interest.

Chapter 1:
"The Cheapest Health Care
is to let them die"*

Mistakes

*Root Canal with pulp
– reinfection
(broke cap right away)*

*Place cap with infection on x-ray
and don't address infection*

*Apicoectomy not at infection
site on x-ray*

No debridement upon extraction

*No antibiotic prophylaxis,
only treatment during course*

No follow-up

Managed Care, when it was introduced in the 90's, was touted as the cure for all medical care ills. Doctors did not know how to keep costs down, so the responsibility was given to the administrators. The problem is that the administrators were given the power to make medical care decisions as well. How a person without the requisite four years pre-medical, four years medical school, and three to seven years residency experience was able to be deemed capable of such decisions is one of the mysteries of the history of medicine. Or, as I shared in the preface of my experience with the medical administrative director, the "cap" worn was that of an executive of "consumerization," and not that of a physician.

The distribution of medical resources according to a consumer model violates the principle of assigning proper tasks to medical professionals. In fact, in the model of Managed Care, whereby the physician is paid a set amount for each patient, the incentive then is to give no Health Care. The pre-set amount is a cap, thus the model is called "capitation." The provider has a strong incentive to ration at best, or deny at worst, Health Care– since providing care takes money out of the pre-paid amount. Managed Care capitation meant that the physician had a conflict of interest in delivering

Health Care, if the physician wanted to be able to earn her living as a practicing physician.

As the drawbacks and limitations of Managed Care are being seen more clearly, the country is looking towards new models of Health Care. Proposals include:

- Health Savings Plan- proposed by the previous administration in which American citizens takes an active role in deciding their Health Care,
- Single payer model- as seen in Canada where the government pays for basic care out of governmental taxes,
- Two-tier system- as seen in Germany in which different levels of Health Care are available, and
- Piecemeal Plans- the majority of proposals coming out of the legislature, including the recently passed bill which will again raise costs.

I believe in the spirit of "life, liberty, and the pursuit of happiness" as written by our founding nation. The American people do not need to be spoon-fed what is right and what is wrong. We the people can decide for ourselves what is necessary for our life, liberty, and happiness.

Health is a major factor in the perception of

> Figuring a spending of about $4800 per person in the US today, that is a savings of more than $500 billion dollars!

happiness. And yet our founders knew that it cannot be guaranteed as a "right." The wisdom of the ages has always known that Health is not something one can control, but a blessing which one desires. Scripture tells of the wisest king obtaining riches and wisdom and long life, but Health was not one of the guarantees.

I believe that Americans should have a choice in what they want to spend on Health Care. Our system is based on choice, and the belief that the citizen can always achieve more. Therefore, we look to have at least a three-tiered system, one that is basic and may be run by the government/ public or private sector and another with more features. The second can be administered by the private sector and have more coverage features. The third method of payment should be made directly by the patient.

In terms of costs, I have to agree that greed did fuel the escalating medical costs of the 80's. Some physicians were taking to heart the credo of the capitalist society, and thinking mostly of profit. Managed Care has done its share by providing competition for fee-for-service, which resulted in administrative costs being reduced. For example, fee-for-service was spending 41% on administrative costs in 1987. By 1990, fee-for-service was spending only 5% on administrative costs. Figuring a spending of about $4800 per person in the US today, that is a savings of more than $500 billion dollars!

By comparison, Managed Care was spending 32% in administrative costs in 1987, better than fee-for-service when it began, but spent 57% in administrative costs by 1990. We can see how money travels to those who are in the decision-making seat. As administrators, the interests are capitalism and the running of programs. As physicians, the interests are the patient-physician relationship and professionalism.

*The title quote of this chapter came from a friend, a fellow physician who worked at the National Institute of Health and specialized in the statistical and financial aspects of medicine. It is the logical conclusion for administrators, if the first priority is cost under a capitation system. The experiment of Managed Care has run its course, and shown that it is a model for consumer business, not a public Health Care system if we wish to have any public left alive.

Chapter 2:
"Another missed starting point"

Reaction
Osteoma
- nice name for a piece of bone
Not normally part of
The 208 - counted body

- could this be a reaction to
1. loss of bone due to apicoectomy and therefore
merely a mechanical
compensation of
shifted forces?

2. reaction to chronic and
flareups of infection

fact: bone site increases and decreases in size,
corresponding to intensity
of illness.

*ENT noticed increased size post off Antibiotics,
now again decreasing post recovery.
Increase at first– notified me of
raging infection in maxilla.*

Would you want a medical doctor to be constantly afraid that the patient will sue them for malpractice? In other words, do you want a person who is nervous and emotionally-charged telling you what to do or have a knife in their hand? It would be like a person with a jackhammer afraid that he would hammer outside the lines and be sued for $500,000.

If you have ever been nervous, you know it would be better to make that big decision or operate that heavy machinery when you are calm. Emotions play a big part in our well-being. Acute emotions can cause accidents, such as road rage. Chronic emotions are known to be the cause of physical illnesses, such as stomach ulcers and heart attacks.

Many times, the body compensates for the stress it is facing. For example, cortical levels (a normal hormone) are responsible for increasing when we are in the "flight or fight" mode. But having chronically elevated hormone levels is detrimental, and leads to ulcers and heart attacks, and a myriad of other diseases.

The chronic infection in my teeth led my body to compensate also, by having immune cells flood the area. Unfortunately, as it attacks the infection, the immune cells can also damage normal tissue, along with the destruction caused by the microbes (bacteria, fungi, etc.). A hole was being made in my middle facial bone, the maxilla, by the chronic infection. To compensate for the loss of bone and stability in my facial bone where the infection was, my body increased bone production in my maxilla around the infection. Infection itself also causes the body to try to "wall up" the foreign invaders with dense tissue, such as fibrous tissue or bone. The reactive bone growth was called an "osteoma."

Defensive medicine is like a chronic infection. It is destructive and detrimental to the medical community. The medical community, of course, includes the patients. When emotions are high, there is actually a higher chance that mistakes *will* happen. At a ritzy private hospital, I was told that the VIP patients were the *most likely* to have something go wrong with their treatment. In addition, the wasted Health Care services and costs to fix these mistakes are like an osteoma— markers of defensive medicine's destructive path.

In a recent national poll of medical doctors, two-thirds of the doctors reported that they are afraid of lawsuits, and therefore practice defensive medicine. The cost of the lawsuits themselves is equally staggering, raising medical malpractice insurance fees for one doctor up to $200,000 per year. When I was in training, a surgeon related to me a story. I believe he was teaching me about the traps of legalism. He told me that a patient came to him and announced, "I have AIDS (Acquired Immunodeficiency Syndrome). Are you going to operate on me?" The surgeon told me he knew that if he said, "No," the patient would then sue him. So he said, "Yes." The patient disappeared and did not bother the surgeon.

In most lawsuits in which the object is to obtain quick money, everyone in the medical community loses. Lawsuits themselves are emotionally-charged situations. Indeed, lawsuits are *meant* to be stressful. It feels like the mentality of keeping your opponents off-balance by increasing their stress levels, a technique often used in battles, has bled into the mentality of medicine.

In legal suits, the medical doctors are somehow the "enemies" that need to be kept off-balance. As a reaction, the doctors practice medicine defensively. Yet <u>both the doctors and the patients lose</u> in defensive medicine. The increased emotional stress given to the patients as they are subjected to the unnecessary tests and procedures is a negative emotional situation harming the patient in numerous ways.

First, the patients wonder if they have a debilitating disease– perhaps cancer or a terminal illness. Second, the time and energy spent going to the tests and procedures is substantial. Many times, the patients are treated like objects in a factory line, as the staff calls out, "Next!"

Ironically, this increased stress can *itself* lead to illness. I have already talked about ulcers and heart attacks. Americans are one of the people most prone to high incidences of these diseases.

These initial drawbacks of defensive medicine are due to the invasion of the business mentality into medicine. The business climate of *battle* is being reflected more and more in Health Care. Business people are encouraged to read books with titles like, "The Art of War."

William F. May, a recognized ethicist, talks about how defensive medicine has detrimentally altered Health Care. Dr. Michael Stein, author of "The Addict," admits to having practiced defensive medicine himself. The atmosphere of legalism has reach *epidemic* proportions.

Where will it end? In Chapter 1, we saw how the business model is not one that translates into the medical field. The business model, wherein insurance companies are paid up-front premiums, is one in which highest economic gain is achieved by giving *no care*.

In this chapter, we examine the dilemma of defensive medicine, wherein the incentive is to give *too much* care. Like Goldilocks in the woods, we feel we are looking for care that is "just right." Perhaps better put: we are hoping for an acceptable middle ground. Medicine is an art, with room for interpretation and innovation. We have come a long way from the days of blood letting. Yet medicine is always learning, and changing– however slowly.

> we are hoping for an acceptable middle ground

Empirical science, meaning the sum knowledge of the detailed information, is what is preferred by physical medicine. Therefore, in terms of defensive medicine, the more details the better. The more tests and procedures, the surer one can be.

Yet as a society, we need to recognize that ordering a gazillion more tests could only increase the "sureness" of the diagnosis by a couple of percentages. That is, instead of being 70% sure, we are now 73% sure. But at least we have exhausted all known diagnostic methods, which must be better!

Actually, the extra 3% may not be worth the costs: in human resources, economics, and emotions. Every decision must be weighed in its benefits and costs, and every treatment decision has both. I am not advocating settling for a 30% surety when a couple of simple tests, such as urine or blood work, can increase it to 70%. What I am advocating is examining each case on its own merits, within the accepted standards of that diagnosis.

Because of the large amount of scientific information available for many of the diseases, there is a more definable ground of correct medical practice. The people in research, the academic physicians, are often the ones who are responsible for gathering the data to establish the best standards of practice. Evidence-based medicine utilizes statistical methods that confer acceptability to study results based on the probability that it is 95% accurate for a given test population.

Medicine, unlike many fields, is clearer in the expectations of the medical community. Clarity is, in fact, good news for physicians. Clarity limits the amount of emotional games that can be played by attorneys in lawsuits.

I once heard a defense attorney speak on a conference about malpractice suits. He said that the best way to fight fraudulent medical lawsuits is to not give in. In the legal community, most cases are settled out of court. The prosecuting attorney knows that many times it is not worth the medical doctor's emotional reserves to fight a lawsuit. Therefore, even if a lawsuit is fraudulent, the chances are good that the prosecuting team will gain some money in a settlement.

The defense attorney said that by addressing each lawsuit, the prosecuting attorneys would then be sent the message that a fraudulent lawsuit is not easy money. Therefore, the amount of fraudulent lawsuits would decrease.

> In the long run, the doctors and patients would be saving themselves from unnecessary stress.

In the long run, the doctors and patients would be saving themselves from unnecessary stress.

At the same time, our health is one of the most emotional areas of our lives. I remember when my eyes started to cake up, peel, swell up, and turn red– I got emotional. I am a very rational person, even when emotional. Most people cannot hold the rational and the emotional in tension. However, during this episode, even I felt the helplessness and pain of the unknown. I understood better how my patients feel.

Fortunately, for me, the situation was environmental. It is easier to change one's environment than to change one's inherited genes. A topical steroid cream and an antibiotic ointment were sufficient to decrease the inflammation and infection.

A topical cream is not enough to fix sleepless

nights when one is wondering if one has cancer. A cream is not enough in the bank account when a family insurance plan can cost $22,000 per year. An ointment is not enough when one has to decide whether to pay the mortgage or the medical bill.

Today's medical insurances have become much more than what insurances were meant for: catastrophic events. Today, the premiums also "cover" yearly visits and outpatient treatments. Can someone explain to me how it is more economically wise to pay more people to manage a patient's money for visits that he can pay himself? Management is not free, and as I quoted in the first chapter, administrative costs can run over $500 billion if administrative costs were only one third of medical costs. In fact, administrative costs can run up to *half* the costs in Managed Care.

With the expansion of "insurance," the utilization of medical care increases. Since one has already paid for the services, one wants to *use* the medical services. Therefore, only in the case of major illness is the use of medical insurance appropriate.

Medical insurance should return to the sound business plan it proposed in the first place: medical care in cases of **catastrophic** illness. Catastrophic describes both the severity and the suddenness of an illness. For example, many people go to

> Medical insurance should return to the sound business plan it proposed in the first place: medical care in cases of **catastrophic** illness.

the Emergency Room because of sudden events, such as a car accident. Yet many people go to the ER because they don't have a primary physician, or for a minor illness that came on suddenly.

I understand that patients cannot oftentimes tell the difference between a minor and a major illness. Many times, patients are just not feeling well. Illness triage, or the ordering of medical urgency, is usually determined by a medical professional.

Physicians accelerate scheduled appointments for people with urgent needs, so they do not have to pay for the higher costs of an ER. Correctly utilized office visits cut down on frivolous use of the ER. The ER should return to its namesake: Emergency Room medicine.

A correctly utilized ER would benefit patients in two ways: lower premiums and shorter wait time. Emergency Rooms would then be appropriately used for emergencies. Urgent care can be provided at a primary physician's office, or a walk-in/ urgent care clinic. The balance of quality of care and cost efficiency would be optimized by catastrophic medical insurance.

Unfortunately, many people who do not have insurance or have no primary physician visit the ER like a routine doctor's visit. The patient is not paying for the treatment– either the hospital, or the insurance, or the government (in the case of federally-funded programs) pays. Thus, the patient has no incentive to utilize medical care in an effective manner.

A patient who pays for his own yearly visit and outpatient treatment **saves** money. He does not have to pay administrative costs, which can double his costs! In addition, overhead is one of the highest expenses in any business, and the encouragement of seeking treatment as an outpatient generates significant savings.

Hospitals are for patients with major diseases. Even then, as treatment options are discussed, other facilities such as hospices may be the best option for patients. As I have spoken with many Americans, they tell me that it is unpleasant for some adults to have the memory of a loved one dying in a room of the family home.

A significant stressor during hospital stays is the conflict between family members when the patient is incapacitated and not able to decide for himself. Many times, a family member has not come to terms with the situation of a parent dying. We as a nation worship youth. We also refuse to look at the elderly, as they oftentimes remind us of our own mortality.

Furthermore, illness is an emotional stressor in itself. Unfamiliar settings such as a hospital room compound the stress. Family disagreements may cause unresolved family dynamics to play out during the patient's treatment, unnecessarily prolonging the medical decision-making.

I would advise people to talk earlier and as a family, about end-of-life issues. As I have stated, times of high emotions are not the best times to be making medical decisions. When the family is together and enjoying each other's company is the best time for discussions.

> Basic issues, such as an Advanced Directive, i.e. the listing of the important wishes of the patient when he is incapacitated, is important.

Basic issues such as an Advanced Directive, i.e. the listing of the important wishes of the patient when he is incapacitated, is important. Does the patient want to be put on life support (ventilator, dialysis, etc.)? Who will be the first and then second designated person, if the first person is not available, with decision-making power if the patient is incapacitated? The items may be customized by the patient, and signed by the patient and the first and second designated persons.

Why do we leave such important decisions as end-of-life issues to the last minute? I believe it is mostly out of fear. We fear looking at death, although we know it is as inevitable as taxes. We fear growing older, and less able to do the things we did in our youth. We fear losing control as we are put in a hospital bed, hooked up to machines, with people speaking in a language we don't understand around us.

I counsel my patients to talk to their medical team and their family about their concerns and desires. Expressing a fear of death is not terminal. In fact, as we address the issue of death, I believe that we are freed from the anxiety of death, and are better able to live the years we have.

Personally, I believe that one should take care of one's parents as their health fails. Dying is a natural part of life, and is better to be accepted, than to spend trillions as a nation trying to stave off death for those final few months of life. A healthy respect and understanding of death would be of great benefit to the community as a whole.

In the past, medicine has attributed disease to a variety of agents. The community talked about an imbalance of "humours," such as bile, blood, and melancholia. Nowadays, we talk about "fighting" diseases.

Modern medicine has reduced Health Care to the battle between the medical community and diseases. However, Health is about wholeness, and the restoration of the mind, soul, and body to wholeness. In order to optimize health, we need to minimize the detrimental effects of emotional strife, such as that caused by the unnecessary conflicts stirred up by legal suits and defensive medicine.

> It is like telling someone not to think of a pink elephant in the room.

Should we make medical decisions by looking at what we *should not* be doing? Should we focus on *not* operating on the wrong side of the body, giving the wrong medication, treating the patient as an enemy in a lawsuit battle? It is like telling someone not to think of a pink elephant in the room. The more one focuses on *not* thinking about it, the more the mind thinks about it.

Thus, focusing on Health Care by making lawsuit's a participant, a constant companion and instigator, in the medical community is asking for trouble. The anxiety of the medical doctors of always worrying about a lawsuit tries a professional already working hard. The anxiety of an environment filled with suspicion and the goose-chase of diseases wearies the patients physically, spiritually, and emotionally.

Medical resources, like all resources, are limited. We should not have to factor in the cost of fraudulent lawsuits. With a high incidence of legal suits, administrative costs also increase with the legal costs in order to manage the lawsuit's effects. So instead of spending the majority of our Health Care dollar on Health Care, the dollars are going towards legal and administrative costs.

Legal costs. Another missed starting point for Health Care.

Chapter 3:
"If I'm a Physician and I can't understand these forms…"

Tonsils
Lymphoid tissue
Filters, traps, kills microbes,
foreign material.

Yet we take them out.

They do seem to become
old,
fibrotic,
And perhaps inutile
and only serves to trap
and keep colonies of invaders
in its later stages?

Are they part of the first/ primary set of
defenses in childhood;

obsolete in adults?

In that case, its removal
is justifiable—
part of the age of frequent
URI*
and into one of quiescence

* URI- Upper Respiratory Infection

In the last chapter, we saw how the law is not the right starting point to address <u>medicine</u>. In Chapter 1, we also showed how the business model is likewise not a starting point for Health Care. In this chapter, we examine the mistake of starting with a power struggle.

I remember one time when my mother asked me to help her with the Medicare information sent to her. I thought perhaps, because my mother immigrated to the United States when she was already 36 years old, she was having trouble with English. As I read the many pages of information, I realized that her English was not the problem. If anything, the English of the Medicare information was the issue.

As a well-educated physician, I can safely say that the Medicare information was not intended to be understood. We all know about the plight of the Social Security fund now that the Baby Boomer generation is in line to cash in on the government program. The same dilemma is facing the Medicare program, and it seems that making the policy unfathomable is the preferred method of refusing payment.

The government

> The government is responsible for fulfilling its promises, such as that of the Medicare program.

is a powerful institution unto itself, when it should be an entity **for the people and *by* the people**. However, when certain entities become so powerful, they are able to turn a deaf ear to the cries of the needy. The government is responsible for fulfilling its promises, such as that of the Medicare program. Unfortunately, we also know that governmental institutions are filled with bureaucracy. Bureaucracy is not compatible with sound economic practices. The government is suited for setting the minimum standards of a program, but not for making optimal profits.

Taxes are the way that the American people sanction the government's budget. The Medicaid program is an example of how the American people approve of taking care of our poor. The poor are poor for a variety of reasons. Some come from poverty, and just need some help to get on their feet. Some have learned the self-destructive habits of poverty, and need education and training. Some have given up on themselves, and need spiritual and emotional support.

The recent Health Care bill under President Obama should be commended for addressing the insurance companies' strategy of "cherry-picking" their customers, i.e. only accepting people without previous medical conditions. However, the administration "cherry-picks" people on their task force panels that have power: attorneys, insurance executives, large companies. Health Care panels should include those who understand the practical elements of Health Care: the medical team.

> Health Care panels should include those who understand the practical elements of Health Care: the medical team.

Yet the recent bill reflects the people *in power* by mandating that citizens choose between a government plan or an insurance plan. Where is the pioneer spirit in which the people have the liberty to make decisions for their own treatment course? Each of the two choices offered by the bill burdens the patient with restrictions and a fixed payment. As discussed in the last chapter, the most economically sound method of payment for outpatient and non-emergency treatment is direct payment. In other words, fee-for-service payment is the optimal method for outpatient and non-emergency Health Care.

In 1988, the Medicare Catastrophic Coverage Act was implemented. **Catastrophic**, as I have mentioned, means that an event is of a major scale and is sudden in its onset. *Chronic* major illness is of a different category, with its own set of dynamics. The government knew that catastrophic events, such as relief for hurricanes, is something for which they should provide the citizens of a country that cares about said citizens.

The expansion of health "insurance" to include what is in reality "coverage" is a factor of a business wanting a bigger piece of the pie. The natural tendency of an entity is to want to get bigger. The same holds true for the governmental system.

However, just as business is not the optimal model for the starting point of Health Care, bureaucracy is not the executive in Health Care policy. Each of these two entities have their place in Health Care reform, in terms of the administration of care. When either tries to become the executive of Health Care, the country runs into trouble.

Educational videos about our governmental system explain that the balance of power is achieved by having Executive, Legislative, and Judicial branches of government. In the same way, our Health Care system can benefit from this separation of interests. Our founding fathers knew that when one wears too many hats, there tends to be confusion. A clear role and expectation of duty helps to keep the country operating smoothly.

Medicare has tried to force the Executives', or physicians', hands by setting up a reimbursement maximum for medical treatment. The insurance companies followed suit, as the reimbursements are low for the amount of education and training that physicians have accrued. In fact, physicians do not make as much income in their lifetime in relation to professionals with comparable education until their mid-forties. This comparison doesn't take into account the intensive training that physicians also undergo, at stressful and long hours, as a medical resident..

It's true that most physicians, even once they have their own practice, do not have the time to organize for their interests in government. I believe in working with the government to achieve the best results for the American people. So after reading an opinion printed by my local political representative, I decided to respond to the politician's statement that Health Care is a "right" of people. I asked the politician if it is acceptable for a "right" of Health Care that the physician be made a

> I believe in working with the government to achieve the best results for the American people.

government worker without her consent. His reply was basically, "yes."

How has it become acceptable to have a totalitarian method of government? Has the people become so negligible in the bureaucracy's eyes that it no longer even considers the basic tenets of our Declaration of Independence: life, liberty, and the pursuit of happiness? Does the bureaucracy believe itself to be God, with the "right" to overrule the wishes of its citizens?

People who do wish for a national medical insurance often point to Canada as a model. Yet one hears of people who have been impacted by a single payer insurance that rations Health Care. Kidney transplants are often one casualty of the program.

A positive point of the Canadian plan is that overhead is controlled. Akin to the U.S. HMO plans, overhead is around 10%. One reason is that governmental plans are not subject to as many legal suits, so that malpractice insurance costs may be much lower.

I believe a governmental Health Care plan can be feasible. For example, I applaud the government for taking care of its poorer citizens through Medicaid. At the same time, I believe that what makes our country great is the diversity and creativity encouraged by allowing free market competition.

Why do we need to limit spending for kidney transplants if the patient can afford the costs? Is it not unreasonable to force others to comply with our standard of living? Each patient is his own decision-maker, because each patient knows best his own values and situation.

Therefore, I believe that there should exist at least three methods of Health Care payment: governmental, private insurance, and free enterprise or fee-for-service. The governmental plan is best suited for providing a minimum standard of care. A second method of Health Care can be provided by private insurance: which can range from just catastrophic insurance to more medical coverage. Fee-for-service is preserved to allow for innovative and pioneering treatment.

> Therefore, I believe that there should exist at least three methods of Health Care payment: governmental, private insurance, and free enterprise or fee-for-service.

Our government should be held accountable for its promises. Yet the people should also know that they are responsible for holding the government accountable. When Medicare doesn't have enough in its budget to cover the people, perhaps the best lesson learned is that we as a people should plan for our futures through investment savings.

Long-term budgeting is perhaps best left in the hands of the people themselves. Catastrophic coverage is the responsibility of a government in which a society takes care of its citizens. By assigning appropriate roles, the payment options are clearly in the hands of the people. The people may decide, at a time when they are able to decide during non-catastrophic events, how and where they would like to receive Health Care.

Chapter 4:
"The Patient-Physician Relationship"

Flashback to another moment,
a senior psychiatry resident, asking me how it
was that the inpatients at the facility
seemed to respond more to my
tending. My reply, "I treat them like people."

A conference on mental illness
pointed to the most significant
factor in recovery from mental disease:
a long-term relationship with
someone involved in their care.

I know what it feels like to be in pain. When I was first exposed to a large load of mold in my student housing, I experienced pain in my sinus that would not let me sleep. As a physician, I believe that sleep is one of the best cognitive and mood regulators. One night's sleep loss was okay, having been trained in my surgical rotations. Two nights and I am very cranky. That summer was the first time I had ever had three nights without sleep, due to pain.

I am not a naturally anxious person. In fact, you might say that I under-react to stimuli. However, once I experienced three days sleep-deprivation, all bets were off. I was engaged in an intensive summer language course, ancient language course, so I was studying all the time, except time not spent on sleeping, eating, and classes. I actually didn't have time to go grocery shopping during this period. This meant that the 1 ½ hours, including the round-trip walk time, meant being 1 ½ hours behind on my studies. I tried, as a good student, to rest during the extra class-time that I didn't need for my "A."

I even tried to get another place to live in. But it was finals, and there was no more time for anything but studying. Unfortunately, studying is one of the first things that I cannot do when I am sleep-deprived. I can show up to classes, I can take notes, I can talk to my colleagues, but I can't study when I need sleep. (Another thing that I can't do when sleep-deprived is drive a car; probably a good thing to know.)   I had a 96 average going in, but had to withdraw from the class by the end of the summer.

The loss of 6 credits of a 4.0 grade point average was not the worst consequence of the mold exposure. The worst was that the apartment landlord had decided to wet shampoo the carpet, after I had relayed the report by the health center that the best course was to have the carpet removed. Since they stated that the carpet was bonded to the floor, they offered to shampoo the carpet.

When I spoke with them, they told me they would <u>dry</u> shampoo it. It was not until I returned to the apartment, finding mold growth everywhere– including my personal possessions, that I learned that they had committed so terrible a mistake. You see, mold loves moisture, which is why it usually appears after a basement is flooded. I had lost my furniture, my books, my clothing, my paperwork, and more– all in the stroke of an afternoon. Not only that, I had been enduring this situation for almost two months now, and my reserve of strength had become depleted. I finally had to salvage a few of the most important and indestructible belongings, and move.

This episode left me drained. I had lost faith in the school to allow such a situation to occur. I was in deep pain, as my sinuses continued to hurt since the only place I could find on short notice was also moldy (of course, much less moldy than the school housing). The fungal expert had told me that if the concentration of mold were high enough in a domicile, then anyone would have a detrimental reaction.

It was a failure of relationship. The school had a duty to provide a livable environment. Even after I had notified them of the mold problem, they failed to rectify it. In fact, they made it worse by wet shampooing the apartment.

In my introduction, I talked about the treatment of dentists that caused me to have a raging infection three inches from my brain for 7 years. Even though the dentists caused me pain, money, and energy—most did it out of ignorance. The first dentist, who did the initial root canal, also placed a crown that *broke the next day.* He did not have the technical expertise.

The second dentist missed the infection on xray; she did not do it on purpose. The first endodontist took the word of the second dentist who referred me to him, without checking out the x-rays himself. The last pair of dentists knew that I had a case worthy of reimbursement, as they had failed to perform their duty that lead to direct damages, and they refunded me their fees.

More similar to the school's actions are a second endodontist's actions. He had the information that I relayed stating that it was a certain root from which the infection was coming. A top institution had traced the infection to that root, which had then burrowed through my face bone to exit the side of my gums. The endodontist proceeded to perform the procedure on the two other roots.

It wasn't until the infectious draining from the side of my face _recurred_ that I found out the endodontist had not taken care of the originating root. He said that he hadn't done it because it was the most difficult root to get to. Did he believe that fixing the non-causal roots would somehow miraculously fix the problem? I couldn't believe it.

What is on the mind of these people, the school administrators and the dentists, when they act this way? Is it greed? Is it the finger-pointing game, in which distraction is the method to help the culprits get away? Is it a fear of saying that a mistake has been made? A mistake does not automatically mean a lawsuit. However, it appears that fear makes it seem like that in the mind of some people.

Then there is the story of my friend who drove

> The patient proceeded to faint.

himself to the medical center, feeling very ill. He had just enough strength to enter the medical office and tell the receptionist that he "did not feel very well." The first question that the receptionist asked was, "do you have insurance?" The patient then proceeded to faint. When he awoke, he sensed that the medical office was not so much interested in his welfare, but rather in whether or not he would litigate against the medical office. We see what this medical facility had on it's mind, first: money and second: litigation.

How **should** the Patient-Physician relationship be? In chapter 1, we saw the detriments of basing care on money; the end result is the cheapest care is letting patients die without delivering any health care. Chapter 2 explored the effects of litigation upon the medical community, which produces a "defensive medicine" mentality. Again, not the way a healthy patient-physician relationship should be. Chapter 3 related the woes of the Medicare population when dealing with a power that can turn a deaf ear if it so chooses.

Wholistic therapy takes into consideration the

> **Wholistic** therapy takes into consideration the whole patient as a person.

whole patient as a person. The patient is not just a purse, a belligerent, or a pawn. The patient has basic needs that lead to health: physical, spiritual, and emotional. Cognitive and social are also types of health, but the general physician, I believe, may be less able to cover all five areas–leaving room for the other members of the team, as discussed in the next chapter.

I define the relationship as <u>patient</u>-physician, listing the patient first as the primary decision-maker. Dr. Abigail Rian Evans speaks on the centrality of the patient in the healing process. She describes how the patient initiates the relationship, decides based on his values, prevents paternalism, and chooses the level and extent of involvement of family, community, and other health care workers.

> Dr. Abigail Rian Evans speaks on the centrality of the patient in the healing process.

I believe Dr. Evans' point for the counteraction of paternalism in physicians is valuable. As is often the case when a person knows more about a topic than another, the tendency is to condescend to the second person. This is especially true when it is condoned by the community at large; the community feeling that such medical knowledge or truth may be "too much" for the patient.

In the healthy patient-physician relationship, the patient is the first person. The patient has the power or autonomy to decide how much Health Care he needs, and from whom he will accept the care. Equally important in the relationship is that the patients are the primary persons responsible for their health. The patient is not an object or a victim, but an active decision-maker. Paternalism evokes the parental image, whereby the physician is the guardian of the patient, and the primary decision-maker. A suspended infantile state is not healthy for an adult. Part of being a healthy adult is to be given the responsibility, and likewise taking the responsibility, for oneself.

The physician, as the second part of the relationship, has the responsibility to fulfill her vows. In this case, the vows were made as part of the professional code, and are reflected in the Hippocratic Oath:

I SWEAR BY APOLLO THE PHYSICIAN, AND ASCLEPIUS, AND HYGEIA, AND PANACEA AND ALL THE GODS AND GODDESSES AS MY WITNESSES, THAT, ACCORDING TO MY ABILITY AND JUDGMENT, I WILL KEEP THIS OATH AND THIS CONTRACT:

TO HOLD HIM WHO TAUGHT ME THIS ART EQUALLY DEAR TO ME AS MY PARENTS, TO BE A PARTNER IN LIFE WITH HIM, AND TO FULFILL HIS NEEDS WHEN REQUIRED; TO LOOK UPON HIS OFFSPRING AS EQUALS TO MY OWN SIBLINGS, AND TO TEACH THEM THIS ART, IF THEY SHALL WISH TO LEARN IT, WITHOUT FEE OR CONTRACT; AND THAT BY THE SET RULES, LECTURES, AND EVERY OTHER MODE OF INSTRUCTION, I WILL IMPART A KNOWLEDGE OF THE ART TO MY OWN SONS, AND THOSE OF MY TEACHERS, AND TO STUDENTS BOUND BY THIS CONTRACT AND HAVING SWORN THIS OATH TO THE LAW OF MEDICINE, BUT TO NO OTHERS.

I WILL USE THOSE DIETARY REGIMENS WHICH WILL BENEFIT MY PATIENTS ACCORDING TO MY GREATEST ABILITY AND JUDGMENT, AND I WILL DO NO HARM OR INJUSTICE TO THEM.

I WILL NOT GIVE A LETHAL DRUG TO ANYONE IF I AM ASKED, NOR WILL I ADVISE SUCH A PLAN; AND SIMILARLY I WILL NOT GIVE A WOMAN A PESSARY TO CAUSE AN ABORTION.

IN PURITY AND ACCORDING TO DIVINE LAW WILL I CARRY OUT MY LIFE AND MY ART.

I WILL NOT USE THE KNIFE, EVEN UPON THOSE SUFFERING FROM STONES, BUT I WILL LEAVE THIS TO THOSE WHO ARE TRAINED IN THIS CRAFT.

INTO WHATEVER HOMES I GO, I WILL ENTER THEM FOR THE BENEFIT OF THE SICK, AVOIDING ANY VOLUNTARY ACT OF IMPROPRIETY OR CORRUPTION, INCLUDING THE SEDUCTION OF WOMEN AND MEN, WHETHER THEY ARE FREE MEN OR SLAVES.

WHATEVER I SEE OR HEAR IN THE LIVES OF MY PATIENTS, WHETHER IN CONNECTION WITH MY PROFESSIONAL PRACTICE OR NOT, WHICH OUGHT NOT BE SPOKEN OF OUTSIDE, I WILL KEEP SECRET, AS CONSIDERING ALL SUCH THINGS TO BE PRIVATE.

SO LONG AS I MAINTAIN THIS OATH FAITHFULLY AND WITHOUT CORRUPTION, MAY IT BE GRANTED TO ME TO PARTAKE OF LIFE FULLY AND THE PRACTICE OF MY

ART, GAINING THE RESPECT OF ALL MEN FOR ALL TIME.

HOWEVER, SHOULD I TRANSGRESS THIS OATH AND VIOLATE IT, MAY THE OPPOSITE BE MY FATE.

Many items are of note in the Oath. Physicians are to enter into relationships "for the benefit of the sick." In fact, the physician's vow upon entering the profession to work for the <u>benefit</u> of the patient is repeated twice, in paragraphs three and seven.

Secondly, we are to "do no harm" or cause iatrogenic damage. Iatrogenic, or medically-caused, damage happens most often when defensive medicine is in play. The medical field does not want to be liable for a lawsuit, so all the guns are put into play, including the big guns that the patient may not want.

A classic case would be the "Do Not Resuscitate" or DNR clause. The default case, when no DNR has been signed, is that Cardio-Pulmonary Resuscitation (CPR) will be performed. The feeling is that, in general, everyone wants to be alive, no matter what the cost– according to the legal community. However, Health Care decision-making, or ethics, in each case should be <u>decided by the patient.</u>

> A healthy patient-physician relationship is based on mutual trust.

A healthy patient-physician relationship is based on mutual trust. The patient trusts that the physician will convey her knowledge of the medical choices available. The physician trusts that the patient knows what is best for himself, once the medical information has been explained to him, based on his particular values and situation.

The patient trusts that the physician's primary motive will not be money, fear, or power. He may be assured of the primary goal of a physician is promoting health, because the physician has made the vow of doing good for the patient. The interests of the physician, of course, will include a measure of earning a livelihood, but it should not be the primary interest in the relationship.

The physician's primary interest of promoting health in a healthy patient-physician relationship is a tall order for anyone. However, the most appropriate person for this role is the physician—not the businessman, lawyer, academic, or administrator.

A patient-physician relationship is a unique relationship. The modern trend is to believe that salvation is achievable through technology.

Technology is useful, but it is no replacement for human-to-human interaction. A vital part of healing is the feeling that someone cares about you. First, one should care about oneself. Sometimes, especially during illness, we need another person to care for us. Sometimes this need is met by family and friends. At times, this need is only available with the medical knowledge of a physician.

A physician is someone who has been educated and trained for a total of at least eleven (11) years, many times more than that when including professional experience. She has the requisite knowledge and skill for matters that may be beyond the layperson. Yet the patient is the final decision-maker because it is his body and life.

In summary, when the patient decides to enter the patient-physician relationship, he is usually in pain. He does not have the normal physical/ spiritual/emotional strength that he usually does, because he feels ill. The patient must be able to trust that the physician's primary interest is to promote the patient's health. The patient does not have the resources to check every thought/action/ motive of the physician.

He does not have the strength to play administrator in the process, by making sure that the physician is pre-approved by the insurance company. The patient is the patient– hurting and in need of help.

He is not expected to know the medical field, and he is coming to receive Health Care in the form of knowledge and physical/spiritual/emotional care.

In turn, the physician is the person who has taken a vow to promote the patient's health. She is the professional that the patient should turn to first when the patient is not feeling well physically. Intrinsic in the physician's vow is the knowledge and ability to care for medical issues. Because the physician is invested in the relationship, he naturally shows the emotional care that is half of the care the patient needs.

I remember when I first visited the dermatologist for a nevus or mole that had sprouted satellite lesions, his concern that it might be a melanoma helped heal me, by assuaging my worries. However, on the second visit when he was worried about the costs of the visit for me, he cut the visit short and I lost a vital part of the visit, which was the emotional care. Instead of being concerned about money, even in the patient's interest, the physician should have continued his primary focus on providing medical care. The physician must trust that the patient can decide what is the best medical decision for himself.

Chapter 5:
"The True Face of Health Care"

Chronic Fatigue

Imagine my surprise
when I saw my old photographer friend
look as bright and chipper as
I ever saw him
Usually, he would be a bit down
a bit layered by dimpled
thick coatings on the skin
slower in his movements
I attributed these improvements
to the attractive new fiancé
by his side
and mentioned this change
"Oh, no," he said.
It's because he had
started taking anti-fungals
as a treatment for

his Chronic Fatigue Syndrome
New evidence and trials
had suggested a link
to candidiasis
and the results for him
Spoke for themselves.

I remember my time as a medical resident, that is—the time during the Internal Medicine rotation of my transitional year after medical school. We were on call every fourth night, pretty average for a resident. That wasn't the problem. The problem was when 3 am rolled around, I'd be getting right into my first hour of sleep, and I would be paged for a prescription for stool softener. Stool softener! Pages are to be used in emergent situations. If the patient had not been treated for impaction already during the day, impaction during the night would not be an emergency. The nurses were torturing the new residents.

Was it to make sure we got the message that the medical residents are the lowest on the medical totem pole? I had already been told by my senior residents that that was the case. Did they care about the patients at all? Unnecessarily groggy residents are hardly the best residents to be making medical decisions.

What has happened to the medical profession? Has the vow to promote health only been asked of from the physicians? Is power, again, more important to those in the administrative areas? (Nurses are usually the sector that take on administrative roles in the hospital.) The nurse is to help the medical doctor treat the patient well, not an independent, self-interested staff member.

Let's look at another sector of the medical field that has become separated from the medical team. I mentioned my experiences with dentists in the introduction. It is said jokingly that dental students are failed medical students. While this may be true of some dentists, I don't believe it is a helpful saying for the medical profession. Dentists take care of a vital area of the body– part of the face! As seen by my excruciating experience with a root canal gone awry, 7 years of destructive infection in one's face is not something to be taken lightly.

Dentists are part of the medical profession, although they are not included in many "medical" insurance plans offered by companies. I understand that dental costs can run high, akin to physical therapy costs. However, I also know that the educational costs of dental school can be 2-3 times higher than medical school per year– that's 40,000 to $60,000 per year. Of course, dentists usually have less years of training so they can practice right out of school, and start earning real professional salaries sooner, whereas medical doctors do about 3-7 years more of training.

Osteopathic students often get the same reputation as dentists for having failed medical school admissions. Yet I have known some osteopaths that are a credit to the field. Osteopaths focus on the soft tissues of the body, in relation to the musculoskeletal structure of the body. When I awoke one day to find my neck "frozen" to the left, my osteopathic friend knew how to release the cramp. When my back was out of alignment, as my back often is due to soft ligaments (my mother could not hold a frying pan in her hand as her hand would double-over under the weight of the pan), my friend was able to align it with a satisfying "wow, that was the most cracks I've ever heard."

The hierarchy of prestige doesn't stop with the medical school admission failures. Surgeons make fun of internists, internists make fun of psychiatrists, and the list goes on. I remember during my rotation in psychiatry, I would try to converse with the therapist on the treatment the patient was getting. I literally chased the therapist around the clinic, before I understood that he didn't want to spend the extra time to coordinate treatments. His was a silo mentality– I dispensed the medications, he dispensed the therapy. Of course, the reality is that I talked to my patients and gave therapy also, in addition to recommending prescriptions if needed.

> Where is the "team" in the medical team?

Where is the "team" in the medical team? During residency, what we refer to ourselves as a "medical team" consisted of a senior resident, an attending, a couple of junior residents, and medical students. Fortunately, I have seen larger teams rounding on patients that included the respiratory therapist, nurses, and medical techs. However, the team still only consists of the specific specialty: internal medicine, neurology, oncology, etc.

I started off this chapter with a reference to my friend's systemic candidiasis. I believe one of the reasons that it took so long for my friend to receive the correct treatment was because the silo mentality affects the medical specialties so that the different specialties do not talk to one another. In addition, the greatly increased information required to be studied for just one specialty makes it a daunting task for the physician to try to tackle another's field.

The need for a generalist that deals with just the more common maladies would be the solution to the silo mentality. Freed of the miniscule details available in each field, the generalist would use his unique ability to synthesize the various systems of the body, and render a holistic remedy.

I remember when I tried to address my allergies and chronic sinusitis, I was sent to the different specialists: ENT (ear-nose-throat), allergist, and infectious disease physician. Each talked about what their specialty dispensed: surgery, allergy shots, and medications respectively. There seemed to be a set schedule of treatment– try the allergy shots, with medications as needed for acute sinus infections; surgery if the polyps or inflammation worsened.

At least, that is what I gathered from the compartmentalized information I received. None of the physicians thought to ask my dental history. Dentition was a second-class area of treatment, and probably something that had not been included in their own trainings. The round of visits occurred during years 5 and 6 of my undetected facial infection.

The internist that suggested the different specialists did not meet with me again to go over all the findings of the specialists. In this particular case, it may have been because she knew I was a physician myself. For the regular patient, I believe a summary visit with the generalist to be vital to the patient's decision of Health Care treatment. The generalist is able to talk to the patient about the relative pros and cons of each type of treatment, having a little more perspective (and distance) from the specialty treatments. The generalist acts as a filter of treatment information to give a more holistic picture of options for the patient.

An example of a more holistic approach offered to me was when I was suffering from repeated bouts of vaginal candidiasis. I'd been prescribed antibiotics for my chronic sinusitis, which then led to decreased bacterial flora and increased fungal organisms. Consequently, I would be prescribed antifungal agents, until the next time I was prescribed antibiotics for my sinusitis.

This cycle repeated itself about 3 times before I happened to be on vacation when the candidiasis happened again. This time, a physician's assistant talked to me about the importance of floral balance in my body, and that I should try finding milk with the normal body bacterial flora that had been wiped out by the antibiotics. He did not prescribe any antifungal agents. I was surprised to hear of this, as I had not been taught this in my medical training, and tried the milk. It worked like a charm, stopped the cycle of feuding pharmaceutical agents, and restored my natural flora balance.

On the cover of my book, I designed the illustration that assigned different parts of the face, the "True Face of Health Care," as the different people involved in the care of patients. I did this to emphasize a more team-like mentality to care. In a functioning body, the eye cannot do without the

> The eyes cannot do without the ears, and the nose cannot do without the mouth.

ears, and the nose cannot do without the mouth. Each Health Care worker is an integral part of true Health Care.

Taking the imagery one step further, we also need to have interdisciplinary teams taking care of the patient. During my medical school years, way back in 1995, we had begun trying to think in terms of interdisciplinary medicine. Each person was a whole: composed of cardiac, pulmonary, gastrointestinal, urinary, etc. systems. Therefore, the medical staff needed to communicate with each other as if the patient were a whole person composed of all the areas of the medical specialties.

I'd like to see further integration by including dentists and osteopaths on the medical team. Each specialty has their strengths to add to the team. This would include the herbalists, the physical therapists, etc. Instead of a silo mentality, medicine must model itself on the human being: whole and healthy.

Health has its etymologic roots in the word "whole." Thus, attaining health means restoring the patient as a whole person. Dissecting the patient into the little silos of specialties may be temporarily necessary to get a grasp on the vast amount of information known about

However, we must also put the patient back together again.

the body. However, we must also <u>put the patient back together again</u>. We must be able to appreciate all the facets of the patient's body and health. We must be willing to put aside our pride and defenses, and work together for the good of the patient.

The physician's vow is to promote the health of the patient. Shouldn't all members of the medical team be required to make the same vow? Shouldn't the medical team be a team of professionals, holding themselves accountable to a professional code? The word "professional" means to have made a vow to the community. Pastors make vows to serve their congregations. Attorneys make vows to represent their clients. Shouldn't the medical <u>team</u> have at least the same standards? Shouldn't monetary gain, fear, and power struggles come after the promotion of health in the medical profession?

I believe **separating the interests** of the medical team is key. Then it is possible to focus primarily on promoting patient health. For example, the last chapter talked about the Patient-Physician relationship, and the centrality of the patient in health care. The physician's relationship with the patient is built upon the understanding that the patient is the central decision-maker.

In this chapter, the next circle of relationship is drawn: the medical team. The primary physician is the patient's primary trusted information source.

The medical team now enriches the Health Care provided by including the integral components that make up the patient's health: physically, emotionally, spiritually, cognitively, and behaviorally.

I talked about the primary physician being able to address the first three dimensions of health, at least partly. The educational and cognitive aspect should be further carried out by the nurses and therapists. Behavior modifications I believe best left to the family and community– however, urgent behavioral treatment may be necessarily handled by hospital personnel.

This next circle of relationship must also be freed from monetary, defensive, and power struggles in order to be able to fulfill the vow of promoting patient health. I understand that financial considerations must be part of a balanced budget. However, monetary goals and the threat of lawsuits should not be primary on the medical team's mentality.

Neither should a fight for hierarchy in terms of power dominate over the patient's care. The medical profession has a vow to honor, which should be more important than any personal need outside of the patient-team relationship. We cannot provide good Health Care, if we are in urgent need of personal healing ourselves.

My psychiatry rotation was the only time

that I was yelled at in NYU medical center. Yet during surgery, which is known for high pressures and yelling, I was appreciated as someone who anticipated the team's need and provided what was needed. In the Emergency room, I remember thinking to myself that the people working there needed to leave their personal problems outside of the hospital entrance. It was hard to work with people that one had to treat with medical care, in addition to the patients coming in.

If we are to be a medical team, we need to take care of ourselves so that the patient: at best, receives holistic Health Care, and at worst, does not get inflicted with iatrogenic problems. We are to "do no harm," in the sense of adding unnecessary affliction to the patient's burden. We know that many treatments involve pain, from phlebotomy or blood drawing to chemotherapy, but the pain involved is with the hope of curative or restorative treatment. Unloading our own problems on the situation only worsens the situation.

In return, the medical team should also be shielded from the more unhealthy methods that patient's use to cope with their illness, such as unfounded litigations. The relationship of the medical team and the patient should follow the relationship modeled by the patient-physician relationship. The patient is the central decision-maker, therefore responsible for the medical decisions. The medical team is responsible for providing the information, and the providing the care for which the patient gives permission.

The medical team must act as a <u>team</u>. Struggles of power and status do not have a place in a healthy medical team. The team, including the patient himself, must view the patient as a whole person, made up of all the fields that the specialties cover: cardiac, pulmonary, etc.

The general physicians are best suited to be in the primary patient-physician relationship, as they possess the ability to synthesize the information with more perspective. The general physician is able to convey the information in a more holistic fashion to the patient, thereby promoting a treatment option that considers the patient as a whole person. With this information, the patient can make an informed choice.

I believe that the entire medical team should be professional, and make a vow to promote the patient's health. The vow to promote Health foremost helps to separate the other interests that come into play in most modern relationships–monetary aims, defensiveness, and power struggles. The professional medical team promotes health in a manner that is consistent with both professional integrity and responsibility.

Chapter 6:
"Our Founding fathers would be proud"

Equilibrium can exist
in many proportions
Witness our class chemistry
stoichiometric equation
of our youthful education, perhaps
left in that period.
One can have one carbon
atom, or two and double the
quantities of all the rest
of the equation respectively
Of course, not all integers
work as there is a
set ratio between the
characters in the equation
and only certain numbers
will give rise to whole number

integers.

So it can be said
of the balance of microbial
agents in our body. The
bacteria, the fungi, the
viruses, and more. One
level of equilibrium may seem
acceptable, yet another with
the bacteria carrying a
factor of "1" instead of "2"
is even more desirable.

In concrete terms,
it may be seen in my
oral osteoma. At level
"3," say, it is twice its
normal size and ulcerated, indicating
a raging infection soon felt
by my corpus systematically.
It is possible that more
osteomas have appeared
as new signals of increased
infectious activity and these
must be carefully followed-up.

In my preface, I talked about the competing forces of the Executive role of medical doctor and the Legislative role of administrator when the Medical Director is asked to decide on the distribution of blood products. What was demonstrated in my training is that when one is expected to wear two hats *at the same time*, confusion and decreased quality results. The quality of Health Care *diminished* when the medical doctor is asked to be an *administrator* first.

Throughout this book, I have proposed that proper roles and boundaries be set for the professional. For any professional, she must carry out her professional vows and act responsibly. An administrator that treats Health Care resources like commodities on the market, instead of life-determining products, is not acting responsibly.

As I mentioned in the chapter on defensive medicine, *too much* Health Care treatment can be as detrimental as too little. To continue the blood product analogy, if one were to give the patient type B+ *and* type O- to an O- recipient, the results would be disastrous. Instead of treating disease like the enemy that must be fought by throwing everything we have against it, we should look to increasing the health of the patient we are treating.

The best method that I foresee to ensuring the proper treatment of the patient is to ensure that the providers' roles are clear and consistent. Thus, the professional Executive is the medical doctor. The Legislative branch consists of the administrators who oversee the operation of Health Care access. The Judicial branch interprets the standards of Health Care in cases of disagreement.

Let us talk more about the Executive branch. As in the running of our country, the Executive or President does not make decisions by herself. The President has a cabinet that informs the President of the many aspects involved in running the country: Education, National security, Policy development, Trade representation, Environmental quality, Science and technology, etc. In the same manner, the nurse, technicians, therapists, etc. help the medical doctor to make an informed decision as to the recommended medical course of treatment.

Executive cabinet members are also given the power of oversight in running the country. The Secretary of State negotiates with other countries and protects the country's interests, the Secretary of Justice or attorney general represents the United States in court and oversee the FBI, DEA, INS, and so on. Paralleling this would be the conveying of prescriptive power of medications to the Nurse Practitioner.

In addition, a famous privilege of the President is to have veto power over all decisions. This ensures that the President is truly the Executive of the three branches. Any bill presented to the Executive from the Legislature can be vetoed by the President. The Legislature does have the power to counteract the Executive, but the Legislature needs a percentage number of votes. The Executive's single vote is definitive.

Finally, during times of emergency, the Executive becomes the commander in chief of all troops. Emergencies include times of war and natural disasters. The same can be said of the medical doctor. In the Emergency room/on the war field and during cardio-respiratory arrests, the medical doctor is in charge and given top authority. During emergencies, there is no time for extended delays.

Let us now look at the next branch of a balanced system of powers, the Legislative branch. The Legislative branch gives structure to the running of the system. The Legislature is divided into two groups, the House and the Senate. Each group has different requirements for election, and differing lengths of service years.

The system reminds me of the choosing of officers for a religious congregation. One group holds office for three years, rotating out at staggered years, i.e. each class year rotating out at one time with the remaining two class years staying on. This process ensures continuity and the benefit of those with experience staying on, while minimizing the overreaching power of the "old guard."

Like the governmental system, the Health Care administrators are the delegates of the country's people who have been chosen. We choose our delegates when we choose the Health Care group, hospital, or insurance company to administer our medical care. The process of the Legislature is methodical, and follows its own set of rules.

Of the different types of Legislature/administrator, the Health Care group is probably the most flexible, as it is often the group with the least number of administrators. A second type, the insurance company has the added load of having the goal of being a financially-growing company to its stockholders. Each group type of administrators has its benefits and detractions.

The scenario of the administrator favoring a "blanket-sale" of blood products reflects the stockholders' mentality. The monetary profit of the company overrules all other considerations. Again, I repeat that this mindset is not the primary objective of Health Care. Providing for the optimal health of the patient is the primary goal of Health Care.

> Providing for the optimal health of the patient is the primary goal of Health Care.

What do we do when there is a disagreement as to the **standard** of Health Care? We then turn to the Judicial branch. Article III of the Constitution basically designates the holding of office for the life of the judge. No other governmental person is given this amount of power. High trust is given to the Supreme Court judges.

In the same manner, the medical scholars, or academics, are the judges of the standards of Health Care. In areas of dispute, the Judicial powers interprets the intent of the laws. In the case of Health Care, rules that have been made about treatment options and best practices are interpreted by the medical scholars.

One of the most important jurisdictions of the Judicial system is the power to decide over conflict that is directed against the United States, or cases of treason. Likewise, the medical scholars can decide cases in which the precepts and vows of the medical professional have been violated. Medicine, or healing, is the system that must be protected.

In the United States, one of the highest ideals is the preservation of freedom or liberty. Our country was founded on the principle that each person has the freedom of choice through representation. When our forefathers were not given a choice about taxes, a new country was born.

When the citizens are not given the choice of how they would like to pay for their Health Care services, we should also resist. A balance of power includes a variety of choices. At least three choices of payment should be available: direct or fee-for-service, a third-party insurance, or payment already made through our taxes. The three-fold balance of power reflects the healthy balance of power between the Executive, Legislative, and Judicial branches.

> At least three choices of payment should be available: direct or fee-for-service, a third-party insurance, or payment already made through our taxes.

How does a balanced system of power work in the context of Health Care First, the patient-physican relationship is the central governing body. In this case, the patient is the Executive, with the medical doctor serving as the executive of the professional team. Perhaps the medical doctor can be said to be the Secretary of the patient.

When the patient is incapacitated, the decision-making power is transferred to the patient's previously chosen designate. In some cases, if there is a strong and understanding relationship with the medical doctor, the designate may be a medical professional. According to our societal law, there is a hierarchy of family members that are given the power of decision-making in cases in which the patient has not previously chosen his Health Care designate.

In most cases, the decision is made by the patient, with information provided by the patient's primary medical doctor. Because of the professional relationship between the patient and the medical team, the medical team is part of the Executive team. Each member of the team acts as a subgroup or Cabinet member.

The Legislative body, as previously mentioned, consists of the people involved in the patient's access to Health Care. Payment is one major component of access. However, the decision to utilize fee-for-service, insurance, or governmental services is the decision of the patient.

The Legislative branch is also subject to periodic reviews by the patient. If the patient is not satisfied with the service, he should be able to choose another representative body as his administrator. Unlike the government, I don't see why there should be a limit of number of terms for an effective administrator.

The area of medical research is the domain of medical academics, or Judicial branch. Each year, thousands of research studies are conducted with the purported aim to find new and optimal ways of providing medicine. The vast amount of information is best analyzed by the medical scholar, who then renders his judgment on the best standards of care.

Of course, there are times when conflicts of interest arise between the goals and interests of each of the three branches. Unlike the government, the balance of power must weigh on the Executive side since the United States of America's value of liberty should be reflected in the respect given to autonomy. Thus, the patient is the final decision-maker, the veto-er, with no countering necessary by the Legislative or Judicial branches.

The only limitation to the patient's decision then are his resources. Resources include monetary, as well as time, energy, and so on. I do not propose to bankrupt the nation by providing every service to every patient. The patient is autonomous, but he also lives within a society.

Society provides for those who cannot provide for themselves on a short-term basis. When catastrophes or disaster strikes, a healthy society takes care of its citizens. The patient is one part of the whole of society.

Therefore, in looking at medical care, we as a society need to look at both the wholeness of the individual, as well as the wholeness of our society. The patient's goal is Health or wholeness. The patient is the Executive of a balanced medical system.

The professional Executive branch is led by the primary physician. The Legislative or administrative branch regulates the guidelines of medical access. The Judicial or academic branch judges cases of conflict of interests between the professional Executive and Legislative branches, as well as cases of conflicts or violations against the medical profession or vow.

Thus, the balance of power in a system is grounded in a model of shared power. Balance is best achieved by separating out conflicting interests, and by providing clear roles for all the people in the system. Our founding fathers shared their wisdom in the making of our country that we as Americans should keep in our heritage.

> Thus, the balance of power in a system is grounded in a model of shared power.

Chapter 7: Therapeutic Medicine

Theory

Braces- to move teeth

plucked out x 4

area of pluck
–- <u>root canals</u>

Reason?

Changed blood supply?

Tortuous?

Occlusion? -blood, other links
new isolated space?

Shift of flora into space?
open for tracking?

Left-over nidus of infection?

All for cosmetics
(my case)

What is health? We all want it– yet there seems to be almost as many definitions of health as there are people. Is health the absence of disease? Or is it something more?

I believe in going to the root of a word and understanding it's etymology, or original meanings. For example, the word for healing in Greek can be seen many times in the Scriptures. As I shared in the Hippocratic Oath, the Greeks are one of the earlier cultures of whose wisdom writings we have preserved in medicine.

Looking at the various occasions in which the word healing occurs in Scripture, we see that even in ancient times the word for healing took on many meanings. Taking an example from a book of wisdom, Proverbs, the word healing is used to mean to **agree** or decide on a matter. A wise tongue is a tree of life and healthiness.

Similarly, the physician dispenses health by the words she speaks. The physician may speak words of healing just by finding out the cause or precipitator of the illness with the initial exam. <u>Recognition of a problem is the first step to healing.</u>

The physician also dispenses health by providing knowledge about the illness and its course. Knowledge and understanding helps the patient come to terms with the illness. Knowledge also helps the patient to be able to make informed decisions about his treatment course.

The physician dispenses health by providing words of comfort and empathy. Emotional health is a major need when patients are ill. If the physician is a believer, she may also provide words of spiritual healing.

A second meaning of the word healing is to be **free**. Implied in this definition is the power to free and heal all life. Freedom allows one to be safe from injurious powers, and to enjoy life.

This second meaning recalls to mind the foundation of our great country. The United States repeats the right to Liberty in both our Declaration of Independence and our Constitution. Freedom is a right that is valued by both ancient and new cultures.

A third meaning of the word healing is **gift**. This meaning embodies the belief that health is not a right, as freedom is held to be in the United States. Health as a gift is not subject to any earthly power.

> meaning of the word healing is **gift**

Health as a gift is one that is freely given by the source of health. People may have various ideas and beliefs of the source of health, but whatever their belief– the source of health cannot be manipulated by earthly powers. The source of health gives out of generosity and free will.

As a culture, we are taught to be thankful for gifts. At times, gifts or presents are given out of obligation in our culture. Yet the intention of a gift is that of a free-will offering.

In Scripture, the gift comes from the one Spirit that is part of God. The Spirit gives as the Spirit chooses. The Spirit is often described as the wind that comes and goes as the Spirit chooses.

A fourth meaning of the word healing is **food and light**. Although the two may seem disparate or different at first, we can see that light is the food of the plants. Plants, in turn, are the food of many of the animals.

We need to eat to be healthy. Medication is an off-shoot of what is originally herbal and natural medications. In fact, many companies turn to homeopathic medications to see if they can isolate the healing properties of the plant or animal.

An example of this is an extract called curare that is used to treat heart conditions. Curare is a natural toxin that is used by some tribes to help catch food or prey. Scientists studied its effects, and found out that its mechanism of action included influencing the cells of the heart.

St. John's wart is another example of a popularized homeopathic medication. Known by local practitioners to help alleviate the symptoms of depression, it now has been commercialized and sold in the health food supermarkets. I myself have tried more homeopathic means in the hope of alleviating sinus pain.

Light can directly be a healing medicine. During my medical school days, I worked part-time as a medical technician/assistant treating dermatologic patients with UV radiation. Specific components of light, parts of the ultraviolet (UV) spectrum, were separated out and given to patients suffering from various dermatologic illnesses.

Light also limit's the growth of mold. Mold likes damp, dark, undisturbed places. Because of the last condition of mold preference, human contact can also limit a mold's growth.

A fifth meaning of the word healing is **wholeness**. Wholeness is a state of being, reflecting our existence as human beings. Wholeness as health is found in the words of other ancient cultures, such as the Hebrew word, "shalom."

In a famous story, Joseph was a brother who was sold into slavery by his envious brothers. While in prison, he started interpreting visions. He became known for his interpretations, and was brought to see the king.

The king's vision or dream was of 7 heads of grain. The word healthy was used to describe the heads of grain that were good and strong. We see here that wholeness connotes or is associated with health and strength.

In conclusion, there are at least 5 definitions of healing utilized by ancient cultures that took health very seriously. I took you through the definitions of healing in order to show the richness of the meaning of healing, and to show that health is much more than fighting diseases.

Health is about a state of wholeness, a state that is a free gift of food and light. Health is a state in which there is agreement and harmony, where we can enjoy life and feel safe. Health is a state in which we can grow strong.

During my many years of medical training, I kept feeling that there was more to health than what I was being taught, more than just a state of memorization and fighting of disease. Intuitively, I was searching for a richer meaning for health. I knew that health was more than defensive medicine—fighting to keep back the seemingly overwhelming tide of disease.

It is not easy to think outside the box. Not only are many factors trying to keep you in the box, those factors are also not above inflicting injury if one tries to climb out. After years of being buffeted by people used to fighting, I heard the call of another voice.

I heard the call of a richer meaning for health. Health is not just physical. Health is not just emotional. Health is not about dissecting the person into "manageable" parts.

Health is about the **whole** person. What happens when we dissect a person? If they are not already dead, they will be soon enough.

We are to **preserve and restore** wholeness to a person as a health care provider. Being a health care provider is not primarily about ourselves, as we see from the professional vow. It is *not* about fulfilling Maslow's higher level of self-fulfillment.

> Health is about the **whole** person.

Health is about the sharing of wisdom, and teaching as we health providers have been taught. It is about keeping in mind the benefit of the patient, and endeavoring not to do harm. Health is about respect and confidence in the sharing of private matters.

I have therefore started a practice of **Therapeutic Medicine™** Therapeutic is taken from the Greek word for healing. Therapeutic encompasses the meaning for healing that is about wholeness of being: a wise, harmonious, and free life; a life with food/light, joy, safety, and strength.

Chapter 8:
Medical Reform

I thought it had been the fact that I always carried my "book bag" (really, my father's old brief case) on my left shoulder in elementary school that led to my shoulder injury. The briefcase was the type typical of the 70's, bulky and big.

The clicking noise had started while I was on my "sophomore year-abroad," in quotations because I believe usually one does the year-abroad in the junior year of college. Sophomore year fit better into my schedule, so that I could graduate in 4 years, even with an engineering degree.

San Diego was a lovely place to be, and the average time for students to graduate was almost 5 years, more than that for engineering majors. It's hard to say if the clicking noise did start then; it may be that perhaps that was when I noticed it. My French boyfriend, whom I had met in San Diego before deciding to do a year abroad in

Paris ("before" underlined because it is contrary to most people's assumption that I was going for a boy), was the one who asked me about the noise, "Qu'est-ce que c'est ca?" or simply, "What is that?"

It was oddly gratifying to hear a series of clicks that could be ignited on demand by a particular motion of my left shoulder. Deep inside, I knew it couldn't be good for part of the body to be making loud noises it hadn't before, especially for the next 15 years.

Finally, when I could see the light at the end of the tunnel during my last year of medical residency, I decided to take a look into the phenomenon. I followed the rule of roughly half of the physicians or physicians-in-training of downplaying or altogether ignoring any medical illness in oneself. For some, this also extended to family members and close friends. (The other half of us can be called mildly to severely hypochondriacal).

On my health care plan, I first visited an orthopedic surgeon, who pretty much referred me straight-away to a physical therapist (PT). To me, it seemed a free pass to a subsidized massage, and I was eager to sign on. During the first course of treatment, I enjoyed the interaction with my Filipina PT. She loosened the chronically contracted muscles that make up the shoulder girdle, one of the more spectacular examples of human anatomic complexity and power.

Then, one morning while I was undressing and pulling my shirt off, my shoulder caught slightly in my shirt, and with a sickening crunch transmitted to my left ear— I felt a sharp, shooting pain. Later on, it was explained to me that as the muscles had not been strengthened at the same time as the shoulder joint was being relaxed, the joint had been induced into a state of laxity that allowed for a small amount of force to overstretch the muscles and joint.

Second round. This time it was an intelligent, doctoral-graduate PT who took care of me. She insisted on strengthening the muscles. She was also able to find the correct positioning of the bone (scapula), as my muscles had forgotten its natural movement pattern in the years of injury and tension. All was going well.

Except. Right after I was happy with my treatment, I was told I had to have a new chart. I asked to have my old chart combined into the new one for good medical diagnosis and treatment, but was told it would stay at a different site for billing reasons. Previously, I had switched to a new insurance plan. After this maneuver by the billing department, I started to receive duplicate bills for the same procedure from two different companies.

I mentioned the duplicate bills to the facility. Their response was negligent. I realized that the PT office was in fact asking for duplicate referrals, when my primary care provider complained that the PT office kept asking for referrals when she had already faxed 3 to them in the last month, and the facility only required one referral each month. I found this out from my primary care provider because I had called her, as the facility told me they had not received any referrals. My primary care physician was upset due to the facility's harassment, and I was clued in to the fact that they were billing my insurance companies in duplicate.

I stopped going to that facility. In researching the different health insurance plans, the "discount" insurance plans did not provide for PT. Now I know why.

Managed Care was the hope of the 90's. The thought was that capitalistic mechanisms, which had propelled our national economy to the top, could do the same for the Health Care field. No one thought to ask if economic gain is the most appropriate model for Health Care.

The above story shows how, when economic gain is touted as the ultimate goal, the means parallels the unethical practices common to businesses that is occasionally brought to light, such as the Enron scandal. Take paying taxes. It is well known to have brought down the great Mafioso Al Capone, but what about the average business owner?

Finding loopholes with expert help begs a close relationship to the manufacturing of loopholes. With the tax system, the type of company encouraged is the one who "finds" loopholes. Similarly, what type of system encourages no Health Care as the cheapest or most economically-beneficial loophole? Such a loophole begs a close relationship to corporate business euthanasia*. In my personal experience, every business person I knew, people who were fathers of medical students, were afraid of their illegal dealings being made public.

Capitation as the basis of a Medical Reform plan? We have seen in the recent bill passed by Congress that people are tired of corporate business euthanasia or business-induced death.

*Euthanasia- literally, a "good death." Used most commonly for the practice of a medical personnel killing a patient, hopefully at the patient's request. The quandary between suicide and homicide is one that is particularly relevant when businesses practice euthanasia.

Most people would agree that Health Care fits into a special category. The uniqueness of the Relationship between the Patient and the Physician is indicated by the word "patient" itself. No other field uses this term.

> Most people would agree that Health Care fits into a special category.

In the legal profession, the consumers are the "clients," as they are also called in business. But this is not the case with Health Care. To move toward the terminology of "consumer" in medicine may seem to empower the patient, but the patient as "consumer" in fact impoverishes the Relationship between Patient and Physician that is key to healing.

We have seen that in order to have true Health Care reform, we must confront our assumptions about Health:

> We have seen that in order to have true Health Care reform, we must confront our assumptions about Health.

1. **As a society, we do want to provide** for those who are not able to provide for themselves, whether temporarily (as in the case of children, or recently unemployed) or for longer-term care

(for example, disabled veterans). Realistically, the best value is to provide <u>Catastrophic</u> care; that is, care for Emergencies and acute illnesses. It is not feasible for the government to try and cover everything medical, when people who are in the middle class are not even able to afford everything medical.

Physicians have long tried to accommodate different economic status by having a sliding scale system of payment. People less able to afford medical care are given discounted payment rates. The U.S. government shares the concern for society by providing Medicaid for those around the poverty income level.

2. **Health is a blessing, not a right.**

We may try to maximize it, but we cannot guarantee it. We may try to guarantee Health Care with legal tactics– however, as shown in Chapter 2, legal suits only leads to defensive medicine. Over-treatment can be as detrimental, or more so, than less medical care.

What we are trying to achieve with Medical Reform is to live our lives with the *best* Health we can, just as we try to live out other dimensions of our lives: family, housing, etc. Do we try to guarantee that everyone will get married and have

2.5 children? Do we want to even try doing that??

3. **As Americans, we have the tradition of a "can do" attitude, one of the pioneer.** Yet we have become one that is heavy with legislation and legalities. Our attitude is, "what has the government done for us lately," which can raise administrative costs to more than 50% of medical expenditure, rather than, "how can I fix this situation, improve my life, live free?" As a general rule, administrative costs of 10-15% is feasible in a well-run medical system.

> which can raise administrative costs to more than 50% of medical expenditure

One basic necessity to be able to enjoy a contented, liberated life is to save for times when one is no longer able to work (age, disability, etc). The government may help the people in events of *catastrophe*, such as veterans when they were asked to serve the country in times of war– always a catastrophe for the individuals and families. At other times, we are to have our own plan for savings: not only for health, but for the basics such as food and housing as well.

Temporary help is justifiable, as society benefits from the altruistic care of those who are temporarily caught off-guard. It is *not* beneficial to give hand outs to those capable of working. We need to regain our pride as pioneering Americans, and plan for our own lives.

4. Teamwork is needed to achieve and deliver the best health for everyone.

The patient-physician relationship is the first building block of the medical team. The next circle of relationship is the medical team, who make up an interdisciplinary group, and includes medical professionals from all the specialties: cardiology, thoracic, gastroenterology, etc. The professionals of all the specialties of the body work together to provide Health Care. The medical team provides Health Care that takes into consideration the patient as a <u>whole person</u>.

> The patient-physician relationship is the first building block of the medical team.

Rivalries within the team are not beneficial. The physicians or professional Executives should work with dentists, who have a vital part of the body: the head, under their care. Teamwork should include the nurses, technicians and therapists. The medical team, in turn, works with administrators or Legislative branch to deliver the best care.

In turn, the Executive and Legislative branches

work with the academic team, or Judicial branch, to set the best practices of Medical Care. Our founding fathers had a ground-breaking principle in setting up a balanced system of powers when they established our Executive, Legislative, and Judicial branches. By separating interests, the founders of our nation helped safeguard against conflict of interests.

As a group, the three medical system branches: medical team, administration, and academics are all charged with doing their part in providing Health Care to the nation, each with their own unique roles.

5. **We need to see Health holistically.**

Each part of a body affects the other; there is a balance. For example, the low humidity climate in San Diego engendered low fungal and thus high bacterial loads. Conversely, in a place with high table water, there is high fungal load.

In another example, my shoulder injury disturbed the alignment of not only my shoulder, but of my neck, and of my jaw, and of my teeth alignment. Our bodies are all connected, as the song goes: "the hip bone is connected to the thigh bone, the thigh bone is connected to the leg bone..." I do not believe that connections are intrinsically facetious, but rather hope that these illustrations connect the reader to the need for Therapeutic Medicine™.

Wholistic therapy takes into account not only our physical body, but the integration of our emotional and spiritual parts as well. <u>Therapeutic Medicine</u>™ emphasizes a restoration of the body to wholeness. Each part of our body is valued and integral to our best functioning.

Chapter 9:
"Do I want this Professional for my mother?"

When I was in college, and getting ready for my year abroad in France, I found out I had to have a general physical exam in order to participate in the study-abroad program. I was so excited for my time abroad, and readily made an appointment with a general physician. As I was at college, I did not know the physician previously.

All seemed to go well. He did a battery of tests, and declared me sound. Then I received the bill for the exam.

I brought the bill to the physician to ask about all the charges on the bill. He could see I was upset, and his question was: "don't you have insurance?" I think I started to cry because I wasn't sure.

He then proceeded to take the charges off for the unnecessary tests he had performed: audiology or ear test (something I remember getting almost every year by my school nurse) and so on. Although he had been compassionate enough to take off the charges, the experience left me with a bad taste in my mouth.

This experience was one of the few bad experiences I have had as a patient of a physician. As I've related, more often it has been those providers dealing with my root canal that have been problematic. However, even that one experience stays in my memory as a strong impression.

What then are we to look for in selecting a professional medical provider? I propose that at least 3 criteria be met for selecting a professional medical provider:

A. Knowledge
B. Compassion
C. Experience

Knowledge

First, let us look at the knowledge component. There is a reason that medical education encompasses 8 years after high school– there is a mountain of medical information that a physician must learn. The first years cover general biology: biochemistry, organic chemistry, microbiology, etc. The fifth and sixth years continue the classroom teaching: histology, pathology, anatomy, neuroscience, etc.

The seventh and eighth years introduce clinical work, with rotations through: surgery, medicine, obstetrics/gynecology, pediatrics, etc. Training lasts for another 3-7 years: in the specialty of pathology it is an additional 5 years training, in the specialty of neurosurgery it is an additional 7 years training, etc.

Of course, the length of educational training varies according to the depth of knowledge needed for the profession. For example, a licensed nurse can do 2 years after high school for an associates degree, and then about 1-2 years of education for professional licensing. A therapist would have another set of requirements, usually about 2 years of education after 4 years of college and hours of required professional training.

As I mentioned in Chapter 4, the Patient-Physician Relationship, the patient looks to the physician to provide medical information. Much of what the patient is paying for is knowledge. Accurate and timely knowledge is key in helping the patient be able to make an informed decision.

Knowledge also encompasses the ability to perform specific treatments. For example, the surgeon is trained for at least 5 years after medical school in order to master this set of skills. A radiation-oncologist learns to manage the treatment of chemotherapy. A pathologist trains for at least

5 years after medical school in order to be able to diagnose a patient's illness based on samples taken from the patient.

Compassion

Next, a professional medical provider needs to have compassion. A provider cannot have lived through every illness that a patient may be going through. Therefore, compassion is needed for the provider to be there emotionally with patients when they are suffering.

Passion's word-root means to suffer. Compassion is suffering with someone. The feeling that you are not alone is one that is very healing.

Emotional health plays a big role in the treatment course. Many times, if the illness is chronic, the patient has exhausted his normal avenues of compassion: his family and friends. The professional medical provider is his next resource to obtaining emotional healing.

I am a strong proponent of returning to the physician or professional medical provider with "bed-side manners." The habit of taking the time to listen to a patient is more than a formality, or a means of recruiting patients. The time taken to listen is itself therapeutic.

Experience

Finally, experience plays a nuanced role in

selecting a professional medical provider. On the one hand, experience may be negatively impacting—as in the case of defensive medicine. A professional medical provider may have been involved in a legal suit, and his subsequent interactions with patients is colored by his negative association with a belligerent patient or attorney.

Oftentimes, experience is a positive attribute, rounding out information learned during medical education and training. Medical knowledge is always expanding, and the diligent professional medical provider will continue to read and learn on her own. A patient would be wise to select a professional medical provider that takes responsibility and satisfaction in her work.

Chapter 10:
Poems

I am, that is
My body, a living
Laboratory
for the study
of various forces
        This microbial world
-bacterial,
viral,
    fungal,
etc.

This delicate micro-balance
of physical, emotional,
mental, social, spiritual
Health.

It mirrors
the delicate balance

of services
(i.e. care),
administration,
research, teaching,
and monetary/financial gain.

In researching HCR
     I have been side-tracked

  By the details
    infighting
       polemical viewpoints

Now I return
  to my center
     my focus

of Reform

modeling balance of powers
       As US was established
       Admin- M.D. - academician

& personal stories

  personal themes
     To spotlight

SD: *semi-desert*
4th year, winter
beginning of chronic sinus
infections

--because too little humidity
---too little fungus??

protective factor

balance

- always think of
remember
take into equation

Flash-forward
place
with
High table water
--too much fungus!
(too little bacteria)
Balance

Acknowledgements

I am so thankful for all the people who believed in me:

My friend Jonathan Crooms who had the patience to read my early writing drafts;

My colleague Dr. Torigian who has always encouraged me to write the book, even when I was beyond fatigue;

My site director in pastoral care, Chaplain Ciampa, who has been a rock of support for me and for all those under him at University of Pennsylvania;

My professor Dr. Evans, who taught me so much about caring and medical ethics.

I would also like to thank the people at AuthorHouse for theirs support, and especially

Susan Franklin for her detail-oriented and helpful manner.

Of course, none of this would have been possible without all my teachers and mentors in Medicine along the way:

Dr. Bogart,

Dr. Grieco,

Dr. Simsir,

Dr. Sidhu,

Dr. Witkovsky,

Dr. Miller,

Dr.s Levine,

And so many others: Thank you!

And now, I'd like to thank the readers of The <u>TRUE Face of Health Care Reform: A Physician and Patient's Perspective</u> for taking the time to read about, reflect on, and hopefully become involved in this very important topic.

References:

Clyne, John; Woolhandler, Steffie; and Himmelstein, David. *The Rational Option for a National Health Program.* Stony Creek: The Pamphleteer's Press, 1995.

Evans, Abigail Rian. *Redeeming Marketplace Medicine: A Theology of Health Care.* Cleveland: The Pilgrim Press, 1999.

Goodrich, Edward and Kohlenberger, John. *The Strongest NIV Exhaustive Concordance.* Grand Rapids: Zondervan, 1999.

The Holy Bible: Containing the Old and New Testaments. NASB. Nashville: World Publishing, 1995.

Konner, Melvin. *Dear America, a concerned doctor wants you to know about health reform.*

Reading: Addison-Wesley Publishing Company, 1993.

May, William F. *The Physician's Covenant: Images of the Healer in Medical Ethics*. Philadelphia: Westminster Press, 1983.

Navarro, Vicente. *Dangerous to Your Health: Capitalism in Health Care*. New York: Monthly Review Press, 1993.

Quadagno, Jill. *One Nation Uninsured: Why the US Has No National Health Insurance*. NY: Oxford University Press, 2005.

Shaviro, Daniel. *Who Should Pay for Medicare?* Chicago: University of Chicago Press,2004.

Starr, Paul. *The Logic of Health Care Reform*. Knoxville: Whittle Direct Books, 1992.

Stein, Michael. *The Addict*. New York: William Morrow, 2009.

Understanding Government: The Executive Branch. Thousand Oaks: Goldhill Video, 2000.

Understanding Government: The Judicial Branch. Thousand Oaks: Goldhill Video, 2000.

Understanding Government: The Legislative Branch. Thousand Oaks: Goldhill Video, 2000.